5-Day Psoriasis Natural Healing Program

Psoriasis Home-Spa Treatment Program Using Homemade Recipes

By Douglas Whetstone

ISBN-13: 978-1500953348

ISBN-10: 1500953342

Chapter 1 – Introduction

Congratulations on your desire to use easy-to-find, natural ingredients to treat your psoriasis in the 5-day program! This book provides necessary information about natural remedies that work to treat psoriasis. By following this intense treatment program, you'll start seeing positive results usually within a couple of days. The treatment program is a holistic method of healing psoriasis that involves more than just applying ointments or shampoos. The program includes other critical areas of treatment such as diet and stress relief in order to heal the inside and outside of your body. When all of the treatments are undergone at the same time, such as with the 5-day program, success is almost inevitable. That's why the 5-day program is so powerful!

As the creator of six psoriasis websites and blogs, I have spent a long time researching psoriasis and learning from readers about various treatments. I was somewhat startled to learn that most people with psoriasis don't know much about the disease and how to successfully treat their symptoms. It is common to hear of people who rush to the store to buy a medicated shampoo and don't understand why it doesn't immediately alleviate their symptoms. However, when psoriasis patients use a holistic approach and attack the disease both internally and externally with natural ingredients, the results are quite profound. This book is a culmination of successes that people like you have used to beat this annoying disease.

The program involves a highly concentrated and rigorous program of activities that fight psoriasis, including natural moisturizers, natural shampoos, consumption of psoriasis-fighting foods and oils, stress-fighting activities, and other acts to beat psoriasis. All of the treatment areas are equally important and should be accomplished at the same time.

The 5-day program is most intensive on the first two days. So, it is a good idea to begin your treatment on a weekend when you're not working. Most people enjoy the 5-day program since it resembles a spa getaway while at the same time healing psoriasis. If you haven't pampered yourself to spa-like treatment in a while, you're in for a real treat.

If your symptoms haven't disappeared by the end of the program, just repeat the program. After your outbreak is controlled and disappears, you'll want to incorporate an anti-psoriasis lifestyle into your regular daily routine.

The recipes included in this book can be created from household products, food, and cooking (or otherwise edible) oils that you might already have in your house. If you don't have them, simply buy the ingredients at a local or online store and you'll be ready to start making your own remedies. If you want to purchase your ingredients online, I recommend using the links in our chapter called Online Shopping. Please read the entire book before shopping for your ingredients, as you'll find some of the ingredients, such as cooking oils, can be swapped out for ones that you more prefer.

Warning!

It's always recommended that you consult with your doctor before embarking on any psoriasis treatment or exercise program, especially if you are using any medication on a regular basis. The author is not responsible for any injuries or accidents as a result of your participation in this program.

All of the oils used in the program, both internally and externally, are cooking or otherwise edible oils. To not use oils marketed as fragrances as these may not be edible and dangerous when swallowed or placed on your skin.

How to Use This Book

For best results with the 5-day program, read the entire book before starting your program. While it's tempting to jump ahead to the recipes and details of the program, it is essential that you fully understand all aspects of the program by first reading all of the chapters.

After you have read the entire book, go back to the 5-day program chapter, whether you are going to do the regular psoriasis program or the scalp psoriasis program, and make your food and other recipe choices. For example, for one recipe you might choose to use a different oil than the one specified in the recipe. The book provides many substitutes for most of the recipes. After you make your list and buy your supplies, you're ready to begin the 5-day program.

Chapter 2 - Is Psoriasis Curable?

One of the first questions people ask after they realize they have psoriasis is whether or not psoriasis is curable. Some people successfully control their psoriasis and after only one outbreak, they never experience another symptom. Some people go years without seeing additional symptoms, while others experience several outbreaks each year. Those who are not successful in treating their psoriasis outbreaks usually only relied on a topical solution or shampoo. However, following an intensive program such as our 5-day Natural Psoriasis Healing Program is the most effective treatment plan because the program addresses all of the areas needed to control or alleviate psoriasis.

There are many factors that affect successful treatment of psoriasis. The best ointment, lotion or shampoo for someone else might not help you at all. This is because topical solutions are only part of the healing process. The best treatment for psoriasis is one that involves a proper anti-psoriasis diet, exercise, absence or control of excessive stress, and a moisturizer or shampoo.

Nature provides some of the best treatments which have been used for many years and provided many people with relief. Using natural products should always be your first choice before considering a commercial product made with unnatural and possibly harmful chemicals. It's hard for the average consumer to know which of the chemicals could be harmful for your body, even though their names are listed on the product's label.

Douglas Whetstone

Chapter 3 – Program Overview

If you want to alleviate your symptoms quickly, then it is imperative that you stick to your 5-day natural healing program. Listed below are some proven guidelines, which are the foundations of the program that will help you through your psoriasis outbreak to get rid of your symptoms.

Stay Moisturized

Staying moisturized is probably the biggest aid to controlling the flaking, itchiness, and spread of psoriasis. Psoriasis triggers an accelerated growth in some areas of the skin. Using moisturizers in our recipe chapter will keep the psoriasis plaques moist and control itching. The psoriasis will not completely go away with mere moisturizers, but you will be less inclined to scratch and pick at your skin by using them.

Remove the Crust

Crusty skin almost always covers psoriasis plaques. After the crust is softened by lotions or creams, it can be safely removed. Refrain from constantly picking at the skin and only attempt to get rid of the crust by gently removing it with your fingers or by rinsing.

Gently peeling or rinsing the crusty area after it's been moisturized is recommended but be careful not to peel so much that the skin feels raw. Consult with your physician or dermatologist for more specific instructions on how to do this without damaging the skin.

By removing the crusty skin, the topical agents in our recipes will be more effective. Our topical agents (moisturizers, treatments and shampoos) will help slow the accelerated skin growth and inflammation of your skin.

Sunlight

Short, but consistent, exposure to sunlight can help reduce psoriasis, and is also great for your overall health because the sunlight stimulates the natural production of vitamin D in your body. Some patients have reported great success with ultraviolet light therapies. However, as with all possible treatments you might consider, always check with your physician before attempting ultraviolet light therapy. Over exposure to sunlight or ultraviolet light can be harmful to the skin.

External versus Internal Treatment

External treatment of psoriasis, such as applying one of our moisturizers to the skin, is valuable to the healing process, but internal treatment is more important! So, take good care of yourself, inside and out. It is widely known that uncontrolled stress can ruin your body and can impede the alleviation of psoriasis. Eat foods that are good for treating psoriasis, such as those that contain antioxidants like fresh fruits and vegetables. Stay away from foods that are known to cause psoriasis outbreaks, such as tomatoes and eggplant.

Various Treatment Plans

While most psoriasis patients find a treatment that helps them, the success of individual treatments may or may not work for you. It is common for sufferers to switch psoriasis treatments until they find one that works. There is also no guarantee that the treatment plan that works now will work for you when you have your next psoriasis outbreak. Try to be patient and know that you will discover what works best for you.

Douglas Whetstone

Chapter 4 – The "Powerful-Four" Natural Ingredients

The most powerful and remarkable natural compounds to treat psoriasis are apple cider vinegar, aloe vera, butter (shea or cocoa), and various oils. This chapter looks at the importance and benefits of these natural substances, and why they are used throughout the 5-day program.

Apple Cider Vinegar

If a psoriasis patient was stranded on an island and could only have one ingredient to treat their skin, most people would choose apple cider vinegar. Many people that have used it praise it as a magical solution to treat their psoriasis. It can be used directly on the skin to relieve itching and loosen scales. It can also be diluted in a tab of bath water, which provides a wonderful soaking and cleansing experience. It can be used for scalp psoriasis as a shampoo and/or a rinse. Drinking diluted apple cider vinegar acts as a great flush and cleanser for the liver, which allows the liver to function better in fighting psoriasis.

Why is apple cider vinegar so effective? It's simple. Apple cider vinegar alters the skin's pH level to make it more acidic. The more acidic your psoriasis-affected skin is, the less irritation and itchiness you feel.

Throughout the 5-day program, you'll need to frequently spray an apple cider vinegar solution on the psoriasis outbreak area, whether it's on the skin or scalp. Use this spray solution anytime to relieve itching or when the psoriasis patch is dry.

To make the solution, mix one part of vinegar with three parts of water or use it at full strength. Place the solution in a spray bottle. To use the solution, spray the mixture onto the patch of psoriasis. Leave the mixture on for at least five minutes and then rinse with lukewarm water until all of the solution is washed out. In addition, some people report that they spray their psoriasis-affected areas before they go to sleep. Then they rinse it off the next morning.

Try adding coconut oil to your Apple Cider Vinegar solution, as this will take away some of the strong smell of vinegar. Be aware that when you place vinegar on a psoriasis patch, it will sting!

It is important to note that apple juice and apple cider don't have healing qualities and can't be used as a substitute for apple cider vinegar.

Aloe Vera

Aloe vera is a common and popular ingredient in the psoriasis home remedy recipes. Civilization has known for centuries that aloe vera has seemingly mysterious healing properties to help cure a variety of skin disorders. Its effective treatment of psoriasis is no exception. There are some aloe vera lotions and gels on the market, but many times they don't contain large quantities of aloe vera and are subsequently not very effective. We'll show you how to use this medicinal plant correctly in our recipe chapter.

Butters

The most effective and popular moisturizing creams contain many of the same ingredients, and for good reason. The best cream for Psoriasis should contain a thick moisturizing butter, like shea butter or cocoa butter, which acts as the base ingredient of the cream that alleviates itching and soreness.

Oils

Other main ingredients in moisturizers are specific oils that have anti-inflammatory, anti-bacterial, and soothing qualities. These oils, which are the best ingredients to relieve itching, are coconut oil, olive oil, almond oil, mineral oil, vegetable oil, peanut oil, peppermint oil, sunflower oil, sesame oil, lavender oil, and avocado oil.

Douglas Whetstone

Chapter 5 - Diet for Treating Psoriasis

One's diet is very important to arresting a psoriasis outbreak, yet it's one of the most over looked aspect in most treatment plans. All of the creams, lotions, and shampoos in the world may not help you if you continue to eat the wrong foods.

Adhering to a proper diet for psoriasis is absolutely essential. Psoriasis is an autoimmune deficiency disorder that begins internally, before scales and lesions appear on the skin. Therefore, it only makes sense that internal and external treatments are necessary for effective treatment. Here are some diet suggestions for you.

The 5-day program will explain which foods to stay away from and which foods will help to control your psoriasis. Below is an overview of the main dieting concepts.

Low-fat, Low-Calorie and Whole Foods Diet. You must eat a low-fat and low-calorie diet to reduce psoriasis. You should start off trying a daily diet of 800 to 1,000 calories and then gradually increase your daily intake to 1,200 calories. Eating good, whole foods will also help reduce your weight. Being overweight makes the condition harder to control and uncomfortable.

Antioxidants. Eating a lot of fruits and vegetables is very important when treating psoriasis. The best antioxidant vegetables include broccoli, garlic, onions, cabbage, and cauliflower. Also, berries are powerful antioxidants, especially the darker berries.

Coconut oil is extremely beneficial in treating psoriasis, both externally and internally. Try to consume up to 5 teaspoons per day.

Apple Cider Vinegar Cleanser Recipe. Mix 1 tablespoon with one cup of water. It's recommended to drink this mixture three times a day, at least a half hour before eating. If the drink is too tart for your taste, simply add some honey or some of your favorite herbal tea. Do whatever you need to do in order to consume three tablespoons of apple cider vinegar per day. Apple cider vinegar keeps your pH in a stable state and is said to help cleanse your liver. The vinegar helps to slow the overproduction of skin cells. Some people claim that drinking this formula is the most important psoriasis treatment.

Whole grains are beneficial in your diet.

Lean cuts white meat (chicken or turkey) and fish. Try to reduce eating red meat as much as possible.

Garlic. This is a natural antibiotic that has been used to treat illnesses for thousands of years. What makes it so useful in treating psoriasis? Garlic contains an inhibitor called lipoxygenase, which slows inflammation. It also helps boost your immune system.

Olive Oil. There are many health benefits with olive oil. It's a favorite of most psoriasis patients and should be a staple in your diet to fight psoriasis.

Omega-3 Fatty Acids. Omega-3's are good fats often found in salmon and other fish. They help reduce inflammation and are a great antioxidant.

Turmeric is a very effective anti-inflammatory and antioxidant. So, try adding this spice to your diet.

Nuts and chocolate are highly recommended.

Drink a lot of water. This goes without saying. Cleansing the inner body with water is one of the most productive ways to rid the body of waste and to help regulate one's body chemistry.

Vitamin C. Consume ample amounts of vitamin C. Consider a vitamin supplement if you aren't getting enough of this valuable vitamin.

Cayenne pepper helps relieve itching and pain because it helps to block communication of sensory nerves. Cayenne pepper helps tremendously to get rid of plaques.

Stay away from Bad Foods

Gluten – Many people report that after giving up eating gluten-rich foods, their psoriasis symptoms subsided. Gluten foods include breads, pastas and some condiments.

Red meat and other fatty foods should be avoided by most people that suffer from psoriasis.

Nightshade-family vegetables such as tomatoes, eggplant, white potatoes, and peppers can affect nerves and muscles. Many times these vegetables can trigger a new outbreak of psoriasis.

Alcohol beverages interfere with the psoriasis healing process. Some people suggest not having more than one alcohol drink per week.

Try to cut back on coffee, tea, cola, and other acidic drinks.

Changing one's diet for psoriasis can be challenging, but it's worth it to get rid of your psoriasis!

Supplements

Supplements are believed to help heal psoriasis from the inside of your body, when combined with a healthy diet. Some of the more common supplements you might want to try are vitamin C, vitamin D, evening primrose oil, fish oil, turmeric, and mild thistle. Only take the dosage recommended on the bottle or as directed by your physician.

NOTE: Do not take aloe vera in tablet form, as this will not help the psoriasis and is dangerous.

Chapter 6 - Controlling Stress

Stress is your enemy, when it comes to fighting psoriasis. Many people claim that their psoriasis outbreaks come right after stressful events or a prolonged period of feeling stressed. Your ability to successfully control psoriasis is directly proportional to your ability to control your stress. If you follow all of the other aspects in the 5-day program but do not control your stress, it will be difficult to heal the psoriasis outbreak quickly.

Stress is the prolonged activation of our body's freeze, flight, or fight (FFF) response. This response is necessary for us to survive, as it allows our bodies to react to potentially harmful dangers with increased strength. However, if our bodies activate the FFF response for prolonged periods of time, then it creates a harmful stress on the body. Many studies have shown that people who encounter major or prolonged events are more likely to come down with a disease shortly after the stressful event. Psoriasis is one of those diseases.

There are many ways to control stress, but it is not the intention of this book to teach any of those methods. It is, however, very important that you understand the significance of stress as it relates to your fight against psoriasis and your need to take appropriate steps to use methods that best work for you.

That said, there are several stress-reducing activities we have included in the 5-day program, including a few simple, physical exercises. These activities are useful in lowering stress and can be accomplished by almost everyone. However, feel free to substitute your preferred stress-reducer in place of the one's prescribed in the 5-day program. The important thing is that you reduce stress with a method that works best for you.

Chapter 7 - Skin Care Recipes

Soaking Recipe #1

Soaking psoriasis-affected areas is an essential part of any treatment. This helps to hydrate the skin and soften the psoriasis scales, so that you can gently remove the scales. Soaking also cleanses the irritated skin, reduces itching, and helps to reduce the number of outbreaks.

You can soak your entire body in a bath tub or just soak the area affected by psoriasis. Be sure the water is lukewarm and not too hot.

Mix one cup of the vinegar to every gallon of water. If you don't feel relief, then increase the vinegar concentration.

To treat psoriasis on fingernails and toenails, soak them in full strength apple cider vinegar, poured into a bowl, for at least five minutes each day.

Soaking Recipe #2

1 cup baking soda (can also use Epsom or Dead Sea salt)

½ cup olive oil (can also use vegetable or mineral oil)

Don't forget to apply a moisturizer immediately after soaking.

Spot Treatment Recipe

There are two types of spot treatments using apple cider

vinegar: direct application or with a compress.

Direct applications can be used anytime to treat one or more patches of psoriasis to relieve itching. Simply mix apple cider vinegar with water. Then, apply the solution directly on the skin, either by using a cotton ball or by spraying the mixture from a spray bottle. The ratio of water and vinegar will depend on your preference and your tolerance to pain, since pure vinegar could sting depending on how much the affected area is irritated. If possible, leave the solution on your skin for at least 30 minutes.

Compress applications involve the same technique as direct applications, but it is applied to a compress that stays on the skin. This is especially useful at night before retiring, as it is recommended that psoriasis affected areas be covered at night.

Moisturizers

It is extremely important to keep the area of the skin affected by psoriasis moisturized at all times, since this keeps your skin from forming plaques. Some ointments are also good moisturizers. So, don't confuse the role of ointments to treat psoriasis with the need to also use a good moisturizer. The best natural moisturizers are shea butter or cocoa butter, because they are thick.

Pure cooking oils are also effective as moisturizers, such as olive oil, sunflower oil, vegetable oil, etc. Coconut oil and olive oil are the best. Oils are hydration balancing agents, and are especially useful immediately after bathing to lock in the moisture on your skin.

In addition to using a moisturizer on the skin, it is also a good idea to use a humidifier in your office and home in order to prevent getting dry skin.

Apple Cider Vinegar Moisturizer Recipe

You can quickly make a moisturizer by combining shea butter or cocoa butter with apple cider vinegar.

3 Tablespoons of shea (or cocoa) butter

3 Tablespoons of apple cider vinegar.

Aloe Vera and Oil Moisturizer Recipe

This is another favorite home remedy – aloe vera and olive oil. From a fresh aloe vera plant, use about ¼ cup of aloe vera goo and mix it with ¼ cup of olive, coconut oil, and/or almond oil. Next, gently massage it on the affected area and let it soak for at least 15 minutes.

Butter Cream Moisturizer Recipe

Heat the shea or cocoa butter very slowly on a stove until it is mostly a liquid substance. Do not cook or boil the mixture. Next, remove the cream from the stove and let it cool to room temperature. If you want to speed up the cooling process, put the cream in the freezer for a few minutes. When the formula is completely cool, stir in the oils and blend the ingredients well. Once it is the desired texture, put the cream in a glass jar and store in a cool place.

To use the cream, apply it liberally to the area of the skin affected by the psoriasis. The two variations of this recipe are detailed below.

Regular Strength Cream for Psoriasis

3 Tablespoons of shea butter or cocoa butter

1 Tablespoon of castor oil

2 teaspoons of coconut oil

1 teaspoon of neem Oil

Extra Strength Cream for Psoriasis

3 Tablespoons of shea butter or cocoa butter

2 teaspoons of coconut oil

1.5 teaspoons of neem Oil

1 teaspoon of Castor Oil

These formulas can be altered based on your choice of oils. Many people who have psoriasis become resistant to treatments, so you might find that you'll need to alter these formulas every time you have an outbreak.

After you have put your new cream into the container, mark the container with an expiration date of two months from the date you made the cream. Keep the container in a cool place to lengthen its shelf life.

Alternative Oils

Here is a list of oils that you can use with these recipes. Keep in mind that the oils listed at the top of the list have more psoriasis healing properties from those lower down the list.

Coconut Oil

Olive Oil

Tee Tree Oil. This oil comes from a particular plant leaf that is usually grown in Australia. It has antiseptic properties and helps remove dead cells. Use this with caution, as some people are allergic to the oil.

Almond Oil

Mineral Oil

Vegetable Oil

Peanut Oil

Peppermint Oil. Some people claim that peppermint oil was helpful in controlling itching. Peppermint oil contains a natural menthol chemical.

Sunflower Oil

Sesame Oil

Lavender Oil

Avocado Oil

Tips for Modifying your Moisturizer

There are several things to keep in mind if you want to modify the formulas above. First, the amount of butter should be at a little more than half of the total ingredients, unless you prefer a more liquefied cream. Second, while all of the varied oils in the formulas could be substituted with one type of oil, it is more beneficial to use several oils since their healing properties vary. So, it's better to get a good mix of the healing oils.

Be very cautious in using more than 1.5 teaspoons of neem oil, since heavy quantities of neem could cause dermatitis. Further, many people do not like the strong odor of the neem oil. If this is the case, you can reduce the amount of neem oil or add an oil to make the cream smell better, such as coconut oil or lavender oil.

Chapter 8 – Shampoo Recipes

Should one use a special shampoo for psoriasis? The answer is yes. If you have an outbreak of psoriasis on the scalp, it is important that you cease using harsh shampoos and only use products that are specifically designed for the treatment of scalp psoriasis. Fortunately, there are several varieties of natural psoriasis home remedy shampoos that you can use. You might have most of these ingredients in your house right now!

Be aware that home-made shampoos may not lather like other shampoos, but that's ok. For the most part, psoriasis shampoos are intended to relieve psoriasis symptoms.

Remember to check with your physician before trying any home-made shampoo for psoriasis to make sure it's safe for your use.

How to Use a Psoriasis Shampoo

The main reason to use a psoriasis shampoo is to soften and loosen the psoriasis scales on one's scalp without doing further damage. Then, the scales can be easily rinsed away and subsequently provide some relief from the symptoms. The shampoo is more about treating the scalp psoriasis than cleaning hair.

Many users spread the shampoo out to cover all of the hair, while some do not because many psoriasis shampoos can dry out the hair. It's your preference. People who do not wash all of their hair with the solution can use a non-scented shampoo after rinsing out the psoriasis shampoo. Either way, completely rinse out all the solution before continuing. It is a good idea to follow-up the psoriasis treatment with a mild, unscented conditioner.

27

Psoriasis Shampoo Formulas

Baking soda shampoo with apple cider vinegar as a conditioner and rinse.

The baking soda works well to loosen and remove scales, followed by an apple cider vinegar rinse to further remove scales and to restore essential oils to the scalp. It also gives the hair a good shine. Here's the recipe:

Mix one tablespoon of baking soda with one cup of water and mix thoroughly. Store the shampoo in a recycled shampoo bottle or similar container. Use this mixture as you would any other shampoo and gently rub the mixture into the scalp and hair. Let it soak for 5 to 10 minutes and then rinse with water. Next, as further treatment and as a conditioner, mix between 2 tablespoons up to a ½ cup of apple cider vinegar with one cup of water. Store this in a separate bottle and label it as your conditioner.

Apple Cider Vinegar Shampoo and Rinse

Put apple cider vinegar in a spray bottle (full strength) and spray it on your hair as a shampoo and before you go to bed. Before long, you'll notice the scales get thinner until they disappear completely. Most people use it full strength without diluting the vinegar, but some people reported great results using one part vinegar to one part water, to prevent it from burning so much when it is applied. It is NOT recommended to use apple cider vinegar for psoriasis if the scalp is bleeding or cracked.

Borax and Apple Cider Vinegar Shampoo

Stir about 6 teaspoons of Borax into a cup of vinegar. When you apply this shampoo for psoriasis to your scalp, try to let it soak for as long time (up to 25 minutes if possible) before rinsing thoroughly.

Coconut Oil (also coconut oil liquid soap) Shampoo

This oil contains lauric acid, which is a fatty acid that helps to reduce inflammation and fungus. It is a great shampoo for psoriasis because it hydrates the skin and can be used as a conditioner to rehydrate the scalp after shampooing.

Castile (or Liquid Organic) Soap and Sea Salt Shampoo

Apply castile soap and gently massage it around the scalp. Next, rinse with a solution of sea salt that was dissolved in warm water. Don't use hot water. This formula will relieve the itching.

Aloe Vera and Organic Liquid Soap Psoriasis Shampoo

If you buy or make your own organic liquid soap, then you might try this idea as a viable option for you. Mix one part aloe vera goo to one part organic liquid soap. Gently massage the mixture on your scalp and let it set for 5-8 minutes. Then rinse thoroughly. It should also be noted that some people reported great success with using the aloe vera alone first, and then adding the organic liquid soap after a few minutes.

Aloe Vera and Oil Scalp Treatments

Aloe Vera and Olive Oil. From a fresh aloe vera plant, use about ¼ cup of aloe vera goo and mix it with ¼ cup of olive, coconut oil, and/or almond oil. Next, gently massage it into the scalp and let it soak for 20 minutes.

Alternative Shampoo Ingredients

There are many variations of the psoriasis shampoos listed above. Most of the variations with a person's preference in which oils are used in their shampoo, while some people use oils as a pretreatment or a post-treatment. In both cases, most users let these oils soak on their scalps for at least five minutes before showering. In addition, many people found it very useful to apply these oils on their scalps at night before going to bed. To do this, gently massage the oil into the scalp and cover your hair with a shower cap. In the morning wash out the oil.

The list below contains the most popular oils and butters, in order of popularity and their ability to treat scalp psoriasis:

Coconut Oil

Shea Butter or cocoa butter. These two substances are probably the most popular moisturizers, whether used alone or mixed with other ingredients.

Olive Oil

Almond Oil

Mineral Oil

Tee Tree Oil. This oil comes from a particular plant leaf that is usually grown in Australia. It has antiseptic properties and helps remove dead cells. Use this with caution, as some people are allergic to the oil.

Neem Oil. Some people claim that while other oils didn't help them much, they did find relief after using neem oil.

Peppermint Oil or Menthol Crystals. A few people claim that peppermint oil (or as an alternative, menthol crystals) was helpful to stop the itching. Peppermint oil contains a natural menthol chemical, which makes it a good shampoo for psoriasis.

Vegetable Oil

Peanut Oil

Sunflower Oil

Sesame Oil

Avocado Oil

Chapter 9 – 5-Day Program for Psoriasis

The 5-day Psoriasis Natural Healing Program is a short, but aggressive plan to fight psoriasis. It is intended for those people who currently have an outbreak of psoriasis. If your outbreak is on the scalp, then use the 5-day Program for Scalp Psoriasis. If you have had psoriasis outbreaks in the past and just want to maintain a good anti-psoriasis lifestyle, then please go to Chapter 11 - Maintaining an Anti-Psoriasis Lifestyle.

Program Suggestions and Preparation

We recommend that you follow every aspect of the program. However, there may be parts of the plan that are not suitable for you. For instance, you might be allergic to one of the substances or you might have a physical injury that prohibits you from participating in one of the short physical exercises. If this applies to your situation, replace the activity or ingredient with something more appropriate for you. Otherwise, please follow the plan as closely as possible.

The first two days are very intensive and time-consuming. We highly encourage you to devote the entire two days to fighting your psoriasis. As such, you might need to cancel appointments, send your kids to their grandparents, and ignore other responsibilities. Be sure your spouse and friends understand your commitment to this program and realize that you will be unavailable during this time.

One of the goals of the program is for you to stay away from harmful chemicals during your 5-day program. So, stay away from any chemicals that are not part of the program. Examples of harmful chemicals to stay away from include: scented soaps and shampoos, lotions and creams that are not part of the program, make-up, deodorant, dishwashing and laundry soaps, hand sanitizers, perfume or cologne, and other chemicals that are not natural.

As discussed in a previous chapter, you'll need to prepare a spray bottle filled with apple cider vinegar, full strength or slightly diluted with water. Throughout the program, you should spray your psoriasis patches frequently with this solution so that your patches don't get dry.

All meals should be prepared in accordance with the instructions below. If you are a vegetarian, then use a high-protein substitute as you normally would to replace the meat portions of your meals.

Breakfast food - You can eat as much as you need, but ONLY boiled or poached eggs and fruits. The fruits should be fresh (or previously frozen) and not from a can, since canned fruit is usually packaged with a sweet syrup. The ideal breakfast would involve one boiled or poached egg and two whole fruits. As a drink to accompany your breakfast, freshly squeeze some lemons and add some water and fresh mint leaves. Alternatively, you can drink a fruit juice as long as it is 100% fruit juice.

Lunch food - Prepare a lean meat or fish main course, preferably baked. If you prepare a fried meat, use psoriasis-healthy oil, such as olive oil. Make two or more side dishes of steamed or grilled vegetables of your choice, except shade-growing vegetables like tomatoes and eggplant. Refrain from putting butter on the vegetables and try not to over-cook the vegetables, since the more vegetables are cooked, the fewer nutrients they contain. You should drink water with your meal.

Dinner food - Prepare a lean meat or fish main course, preferably baked, but half the size of your noon meal portion. Make three or more side dishes of steamed or grilled vegetables of your choice. Follow the same instructions for preparing your food as you did for lunch. Drink water with your meal.

Overview

This 5-day program is a concentrated plan of psoriasis-fighting activities that includes using home-made natural formulas on your psoriasis outbreak area of the skin, consuming home-made natural drinks to clean the liver and balance the body's pH level, eating healthy foods with an emphasis on consumption of a lot of antioxidants, conducting mental exercises to lower stress, engaging in physical exercises to lose weight and staying away from harmful chemicals.

All recipes referenced below are in Chapter 7, unless indicated otherwise.

Days 1 and 2

7:00am – Wake up and drink a glass of Apple Cider Vinegar Cleanser (one tablespoon of apple cider vinegar in a cup of water). At first, this drink might taste horrible. So, if you need to, you can add a teaspoon of coconut oil to make the drink more palatable. You should drink this cleanser at least 30 minutes before you eat your three daily meals.

7:15am – Enjoy a warm, relaxing bath using Soaking Recipe #1 for about 20 minutes. For shampooing, use one of the shampoos from Chapter 8. As soon as you are finished, gently pat yourself dry and apply the Apple Cider Vinegar Moisturizer to the psoriasis outbreak area.

7:45am – Breakfast.

8:00am – Stretching Exercise. Spend a few moments and do some light stretching exercises, such as touching your toes, reaching for the sky, etc.

8:10am – Walk for 30 minutes. This is a good opportunity to exercise and think positive (non-stressful) thoughts. It doesn't matter how fast you walk, the important thing is that you are walking! If the weather doesn't permit you to go outside, then replace this activity with a light aerobic activity.

9:00am – Blend one fruit and one cup of ice (and some water if it is too thick) and drink it as a special treat while you enjoy another spa-like bath using Soaking Recipe #2. Soak as long as you want, but it should be at least 20 minutes. After your bath, apply the Aloe Vera and Oil Moisturizer to all psoriasis-affected areas.

10:00am – Peaceful activity. Choose an activity that is peaceful and stress-free, such as reading an inspiring book, listening to music, meditating, or watching a relaxing TV show or movie. Don't watch a show that will make your body more stressful. In other words, stay away from horror movies, mysteries, shows depicting violence, or shows that might make you cry. The idea is to let your mind have a peaceful and enjoyable rest.

11:30am - Drink a glass of Apple Cider Vinegar Cleanser with an added teaspoon of coconut oil.

12:00pm - Lunch.

12:30pm – Apply a generous coat of the Butter Cream Moisturizer to the parts of your body affected by psoriasis.

1:00pm – Stretching Exercise. Spend a few moments and do some light stretching exercises, such as touching your toes, reaching for the sky, etc.

2:00pm – Blend one cup of berries or one fruit with a cup of ice (and some water if it is too thick) and drink it as a special treat while you enjoy another spa-like bath using Soaking Recipe #2. Soak as long as you want, but it should be at least 20 minutes. After your bath, apply the Aloe Vera and Oil Moisturizer to all psoriasis-affected areas.

3:00pm – Broccoli treat. Eat as much raw broccoli as you want, but it should be at least ¾ of a cup. Dip the broccoli in a sauce of ¼ cup of olive oil and 2 teaspoons of finely chopped or minced garlic. This is a very healthy snack for your body. These three items are a powerhouse of nutrients that are much needed when the body is suffering from psoriasis. If your stomach can't handle eating raw broccoli, you can slightly steam the broccoli so it is easier on your stomach. However, try not to cook the broccoli too much, since the more you cook vegetables, the more nutrients are lost.

3:15pm – Rest or enjoy another stress-free activity.

5:30am - Drink a glass of Apple Cider Vinegar Cleanser with an added teaspoon of coconut oil.

6:00pm – Dinner. Add one whole fruit to your dinner as a desert.

6:30pm – Apply the Apple Cider Vinegar Moisturizer to your psoriasis-affected areas.

7:00pm – Evening treat. Enjoy some chocolate, hot cocoa or a blended fruit and crushed ice drink. Try adding 1 teaspoon of coconut, peppermint, or walnut oil to your blended fruit drink for added flavor!

Before retiring – spray the vinegar solution on your psoriasis-affected areas and if possible wrap the area in gauze to prevent the area from drying out.

Days 3 to 5 (times can be adjusted to fit your work schedule)

7:00am – Wake up and drink a glass of Apple Cider Vinegar Cleanser (one tablespoon of apple cider vinegar in a cup of water). At first, this drink might taste horrible. So, if you need to, you can add a teaspoon of coconut oil to make the drink more palatable. You should drink this cleanser at least 30 minutes before you eat your three daily meals.

7:15am – Enjoy a warm, relaxing bath using Soaking Recipe #1 (from Chapter 7) for about 20 minutes. For shampooing, use one of the shampoos from Chapter 8. As soon as you are finished, gently pat yourself dry and apply the Apple Cider Vinegar Moisturizer to the psoriasis outbreak area.

7:45am – Breakfast.

10:00am – Eat at least one whole fruit.

11:30am - Drink a glass of Apple Cider Vinegar Cleanser with one added teaspoon of coconut oil.

12:00pm - Lunch.

3:00pm – Broccoli treat. Eat as much raw broccoli as you want, but it should be at least ¾ of a cup. Dip the broccoli in a sauce of ¼ cup of olive oil and 2 teaspoons of finely chopped or minced garlic. This is a very healthy snack for your body. These three items are a powerhouse of nutrients that are much needed when the body is suffering from psoriasis. If your stomach can't handle eating raw broccoli, you can slightly steam the broccoli so it is easier on your stomach. However, try not to cook the broccoli too much, since the more you cook vegetables, the more nutrients are lost.

5:30am - Drink a glass of Apple Cider Vinegar Cleanser with one added teaspoon of coconut oil.

6:00pm – Dinner.

6:30pm – Apply the Apple Cider Vinegar Moisturizer to your psoriasis-affected areas.

7:00pm – Stretch and walk for at least 20 minutes.

7:30pm - Enjoy another spa-like bath using Soaking Recipe #2. Soak as long as you want, but it should be at least 20 minutes. After your bath, apply the Aloe Vera and Oil Moisturizer to all psoriasis-affected areas.

8:00pm – Evening treat. Enjoy some chocolate, hot cocoa or a blended fruit and crushed ice drink. Try adding 1 teaspoon of coconut, peppermint, or walnut oil to your blended fruit drink for added flavor!

Before retiring – spray the vinegar solution on your psoriasis-affected areas and if possible wrap the area in gauze to prevent the area from drying out.

After day 5 – Congratulations! You completed an intense program to control your psoriasis. If your psoriasis has not healed sufficiently, go back to day 1 and start the program over again. Otherwise, move on to the lifestyle maintenance program in Chapter 11.

Douglas Whetstone

Chapter 10 – 5-Day Program for <u>Scalp</u> Psoriasis

The 5-day Scalp Psoriasis Natural Healing Program is a short, but aggressive plan to fight scalp psoriasis. It is intended for those people who currently have an outbreak of psoriasis. If your psoriasis outbreak is not on the scalp, then use the 5-day program in Chapter 9. If you have had psoriasis outbreaks in the past and just want to maintain a good anti-psoriasis lifestyle, then please go to Chapter 11 on Maintaining an Anti-Psoriasis Lifestyle.

Program Suggestions and Preparation

We recommend that you follow every aspect of the program. However, there may be parts of the plan that are not suitable for you. For instance, you might be allergic to one of the substances or you might have a physical injury that prohibits you in participating in one of the short physical exercises. If this applies to your situation, replace the activity or ingredient with something more appropriate for you. Otherwise, please follow the plan as closely as possible.

The first two days are very intensive and time-consuming. We highly encourage you to devote the entire two days to fighting your psoriasis. As such, you might need to cancel appointments, send the kids to their grandparents, and ignore other responsibilities. Be sure your spouse and friends understand your commitment to this program and realize that you will be unavailable during this time.

One of the goals of the program is for you to stay away from harmful chemicals during your 5-day program. So, avoid any chemicals that are not part of the program. Examples of harmful chemicals to stay away from include: scented soaps and shampoos, lotions and creams that are not part of the program, make-up, deodorant, dishwashing and laundry soaps, hand sanitizers, perfume or cologne, and other chemicals that are not natural.

As discussed in a previous chapter, you'll need to prepare a spray bottle filled with apple cider vinegar, full strength or slightly diluted with water. Throughout the program, you should spray your psoriasis patches frequently with this solution so that your patches never get dry.

All meals should be prepared in accordance with the instructions below. If you are a vegetarian, then use a high-protein substitute for meat, as you normally would.

Breakfast food - You can eat as much as you need, but ONLY boiled or poached eggs and fruits. The fruits should be fresh (or previously frozen) and not from a can, since canned fruit is usually packaged with a sweet syrup. The ideal breakfast would involve one boiled or poached egg and two whole fruits. As a drink to accompany your breakfast, freshly squeeze some lemons and add some water and fresh mint leaves. Alternatively, you can drink a fruit juice as long as it is 100% fruit juice.

Lunch food - Prepare a lean meat or fish main course, preferably baked. If you prepare a fried meat, use psoriasis-healthy oil, such as olive oil. Make two or more side dishes of steamed or grilled vegetables of your choice, except shade-growing vegetables like tomatoes and eggplant. Refrain from putting butter on the vegetables and try not to over-cook the vegetables, since the more vegetables are cooked, the fewer nutrients they contain. You should drink water with your meal.

Dinner food - Prepare a lean meat or fish main course, preferably baked, but half the size of your noon meal portion. Make three or more side dishes of steamed or grilled vegetables of your choice. Follow the same instructions for preparing your food as you did for lunch. Drink water with your meal.

Overview

This 5-day program is a concentrated plan of scalp psoriasis-fighting activities that includes using home-made natural formulas on your psoriasis outbreak, consuming home-made natural drinks to clean the liver and balance the body's pH level, eating healthy foods with an emphasis on consumption of a lot of antioxidants, mental exercises to lower stress, conducting physical exercises to lose weight and staying away from harmful chemicals.

All recipes referenced below are in Chapter 8, unless indicated otherwise.

Days 1 and 2

7:00am – Wake up and drink a glass of Apple Cider Vinegar Cleanser (one tablespoon of apple cider vinegar in a cup of water). At first, this drink might taste horrible. So, if you need to, you can add a teaspoon of coconut oil to make the drink more palatable. You should drink this cleanser at least 30 minutes before you eat your three daily meals.

7:15am – Enjoy a warm, relaxing bath or shower using non-scented bath soap. For shampooing, use the Borax and Apple Cider Vinegar Shampoo. (Be sure to only use the apple cider vinegar as a rinse.) After the rinse, dry the hair and immediately apply a liberal portion of coconut oil to the area on the scalp affected by psoriasis.

7:45am – Breakfast.

8:00am – Stretching Exercise. Spend a few moments and do some light stretching exercises, such as touching your toes, reaching for the sky, etc.

8:10am – Walk for 30 minutes. This is a good opportunity to exercise and think positive (non-stressful) thoughts. It doesn't matter how fast you walk, the important thing is that you are walking! If the weather doesn't permit you to go outside, then replace this activity with a light aerobic activity such as slow dancing.

9:00am – Blend one fruit and one cup of ice (and some water if it is too thick) and drink it as a special treat.

9:30am – Apply the Aloe Vera and oil Scalp Treatment.

10:00am – Peaceful activity. Choose an activity that is peaceful and stress-free, such as reading an inspiring book, listening to music, meditating, or watching a relaxing TV show or movie. Don't watch a show that will make your body more stressful. In other words, stay away from horror movies, mysteries, shows depicting violence, or shows that might make you cry. The idea is to let your mind have a peaceful and enjoyable rest.

11:30am - Drink a glass of Apple Cider Vinegar Cleanser with an added teaspoon of coconut oil.

12:00pm - Lunch.

12:30pm – Apply a generous coat of pure apple cider vinegar to the scalp.

1:00pm – Stretching Exercise. Spend a few moments and do some light stretching exercises, such as touching your toes, reaching for the sky, etc.

2:00pm – Blend one fruit and one cup of ice (and some water if it is too thick) and drink it as a special treat.

3:00pm – Broccoli treat. Eat as much raw broccoli as you want, but it should be at least ¾ of a cup. Dip the broccoli in a dip of ¼ cup of olive oil and 2 teaspoons of finely chopped or minced garlic. This is a very healthy snack for your body. These three items are a powerhouse of nutrients that are much needed when the body is suffering from psoriasis. If your stomach can't handle eating raw broccoli, you can slightly steam the broccoli so it is easier on your stomach. However, try not to cook the broccoli too much, since the more you cook vegetables, the more nutrients are lost.

3:15pm – Rest or enjoy another stress-free activity.

5:30am - Drink a glass of Apple Cider Vinegar Cleanser with an added teaspoon of coconut oil.

6:00pm – Dinner. Add one whole fruit to your dinner as a desert.

6:30pm – Wash your hair and scalp with the Baking Soda Shampoo with Apple Cider Vinegar as a Conditioner and Rinse. The recipe is in Chapter 8. Do NOT combine the baking soda with the vinegar! Only apply the vinegar after washing out the baking soda. After the hair has dried, apply coconut oil to the area on the scalp affected by psoriasis.

7:00pm – Evening treat. Enjoy some chocolate, hot cocoa or a blended fruit and crushed ice drink. Try adding 1 teaspoon of coconut, peppermint, or walnut oil to your blended fruit drink for added flavor!

Before retiring – spray the vinegar solution on your psoriasis-affected area of your scalp and if possible wear a plastic cap to prevent the area from drying out.

Days 3 to 5 (times can be adjusted to fit your work schedule)

7:00am – Wake up and drink a glass of Apple Cider Vinegar Cleanser (one tablespoon of apple cider vinegar in a cup of water). At first, this drink might taste horrible. So, if you need to, you can add a teaspoon of coconut oil to make the drink more palatable. You should drink this cleanser at least 30 minutes before you eat your three daily meals.

7:15am – Enjoy a warm, relaxing bath or shower using a non-scented bath soap. For shampooing, use the Borax and Apple Cider Vinegar Shampoo. (Be sure to only use the apple cider vinegar as a rinse.) After the rinse, dry the hair and immediately apply a liberal portion of coconut oil to the area on the scalp affected by psoriasis.

7:45am – Breakfast.

10:00am – Eat at least one whole fruit.

11:30am - Drink a glass of Apple Cider Vinegar Cleanser with one added teaspoon of coconut oil.

12:00pm - Lunch.

3:00pm – Broccoli treat. Eat as much raw broccoli as you want, but it should be at least ¾ of a cup. Dip the broccoli in a dip of ¼ cup of olive oil and 2 teaspoons of finely chopped or minced garlic. This is a very healthy snack for your body. These three items are a powerhouse of nutrients that are much needed when the body is suffering from psoriasis. If your stomach can't handle eating raw broccoli, you can slightly steam the broccoli so it is easier on your stomach. However, try not to cook the broccoli too much, since the more you cook vegetables, the more nutrients are lost.

5:30am - Drink a glass of Apple Cider Vinegar Cleanser with one added teaspoon of coconut oil.

6:00pm – Dinner.

6:30pm – Wash your hair and scalp with the Castile Soap and Sea Salt Shampoo or the Aloe Vera and Organic Liquid Soap Shampoo. Apply vinegar as a rinse. After the hair has dried, apply coconut oil to the area on the scalp affected by psoriasis. (On day 4, replace the coconut oil treatment with the Aloe Vera and Oil Scalp treatment.)

7:00pm – Stretch and walk for at least 20 minutes.

8:00pm – Evening treat. Enjoy some chocolate, hot cocoa or a blended fruit and crushed ice drink. Try adding 1 teaspoon of coconut, peppermint, or walnut oil to your blended fruit drink for added flavor!

Before retiring – spray the vinegar solution on your psoriasis-affected area of your scalp and if possible wear a plastic cap to prevent the area from drying out.

After day 5 – Congratulations! You completed an intense program to control your psoriasis. If your psoriasis has not healed sufficiently, go back to day 1 and start the program over again. Otherwise, move on to the lifestyle maintenance program in Chapter 11.

Douglas Whetstone

Chapter 11 - Maintaining an Anti-Psoriasis Lifestyle

Congratulations on successfully completing the 5-day Psoriasis Natural Healing Program! Once your symptoms have disappeared, it's time to change your lifestyle so that you don't have any more outbreaks. This chapter provides useful tips on maintaining an anti-psoriasis lifestyle.

Food

Refrain from eating foods that are known to trigger psoriasis, such as tomatoes, eggplant and fatty meats. Instead, eat plenty of the good foods and oils listed in Chapter 5, to include fruits and vegetables that contain a lot of anti-oxidants, lean meats, psoriasis-fighting oils like coconut and olive oils. If you eat fried foods, always try to use one of the good oils, such as olive oil. Limit your intake of gluten foods.

Stress

You might have heard before that "stress kills," as this is a popular and true statement. Prolonged stress lowers our immune system and increases our chances of becoming diseased. This is especially true for those who are prone to psoriasis.

Take concrete steps to control your stress. There are many books on the subject that provide ample ideas that will work for you. You'll discover that the better you can handle stressful situations, the happier and healthier you will be.

Exercise

Proper exercise is important to boost your immune system, lower stress, and lose weight. All of these areas are very important in your fight to keep psoriasis from returning. Start your exercise program with simple exercises and walking. Then, gradually increase to aerobic exercises and walking for longer periods of time. You should exercise at least three times a week and perform various stretching exercises daily.

Avoid Harsh Chemicals

We are exposed to toxic and otherwise harmful chemicals just about everywhere in our environment. However, the more you can avoid harsh chemicals, the healthier you will be.

While you can't always control your environment, you can control the chemicals you use. One important step you can take is to use only green cleaning products in your home.

In closing, I truly hope the 5-day program was a success for you and wish you continued success with the lifestyle maintenance program.

Please take the time to write a review of this book on Amazon! I truly appreciate and value your opinions. Thank you!

www.ingramcontent.com/pod-product-compliance
Lightning Source LLC
Chambersburg PA
CBHW051249170526
45165CB00004B/1636